-Copyright @2020 Olivia Schmidt

-All rights reserved

No part of this publication may be reproduced or transmitted in any form or by any means, including photocopying, recording, or other electronic or mechanical methods, or by any information storage and retrieval system without the prior written permission of the publisher, except in the case of very brief quotations embodied in critical reviews and certain other noncommercial uses permitted by copyright law.

WHAT'S YOUR VISION?

Olivia Schmidt

To my family, for always believing in me and encouraging me to chase my dreams.

To my daughters, learn from everything you can, be strong, confident, and kind. You are my inspiration. Keep shining!

-OS

WHAT'S YOUR VISION?!!!

An ultimate guide written by Coach Olivia Schmidt/ Owner Visionary Bootcamp, to provide 365 ready-made effective Bootcamp workouts and a 5-week daily challenge to keep you motivated to reach your goals! Each workout is safe, suitable, and easy to follow. Try them individually or with a partner. Each workout can be modified to everyone's own needs.

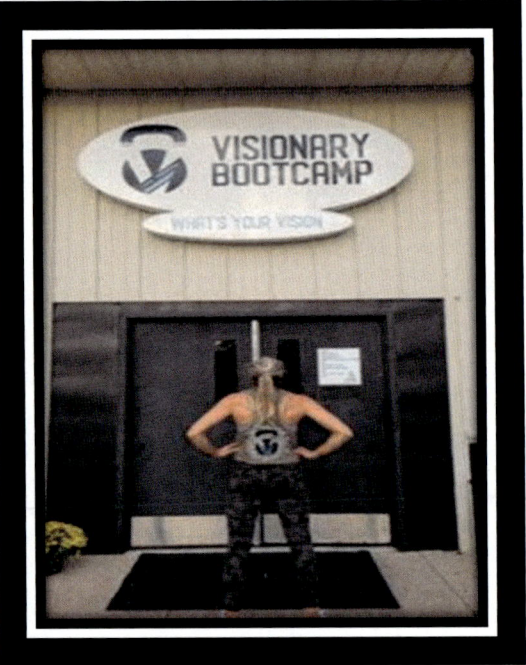

YOUR BODY, YOUR GOALS, YOUR CHALLENGES, YOUR VISION!!!

WELCOME

Welcome to What's Your Vision?!
Are you ready to make a change in your lifestyle, ready to exercise, ready to make that commitment, but unsure how to get started? The starting point is the most difficult and the scariest. This book will help guide you with professionally designed workouts and challenges to improve your cardiovascular, strength, and self-confidence. With the right motivational tools, you can be your own coach. Making the commitment to get fit can be completely overwhelming, with these workouts and challenges already designed for you, it will help kickstart your fitness journey. These workouts are Bootcamp style that combine all different types of cardio, strength exercises, and body weight movements. They push you to get stronger, more toned, increase your cardio, mobility, and feel incredibly confident in your own skin. Each one of these workouts can be modified to your comfort level. "What's your Vision?" is my slogan and for a particularly important reason. Your body, your goals, your challenges, your VISION!!
Few tips I have for you to start your Vision:
1. It is up to you to decide if you are ready for this commitment. Set your goals, but if you are not ready mentally and physically it will be difficult to reach these. NO better time than today! You can do this and know you will succeed! Finding your balance is key!
2. Create a Goal Board. Add magazine articles, pictures, quotes, anything that motivates

you. Put this somewhere you can see every day!

3. Start small, modify the workouts until you feel comfortable, do not ever be consumed with doing the whole workout. Listen to your body!

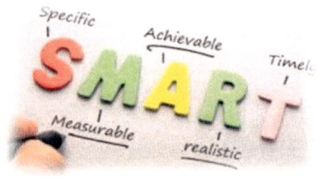

4. Remind yourself that something is better than nothing. Find a time to squeeze it in even if it is 15 minutes.
5. Fear is powerful! Conquer those fears and go for it!!!

6) Learn how to substitute movements and equipment. If my workout calls for 30 calorie bike, but you don't have a bike, substitute for 2 minutes of cardio, which can be running, jumping jacks, jump rope, bear crawl. If you do not have a kettlebell use a backpack stuffed with books, water jugs, use stairs or coffee tables for box jumps. Utilize your home objects for equipment substitutions!

7). Remember proper form is always way more important than the weight you use. YouTube is a great tool to use to check on a movement you are unfamiliar with!

8.) You are going to feel awkward doing certain movements, do them anyways! It does get better!

9.) Rest days are essential!!

10.) Have fun!! We are all in this together. I cannot wait for you to take this journey with me and challenge you with these workouts!

Author Bio

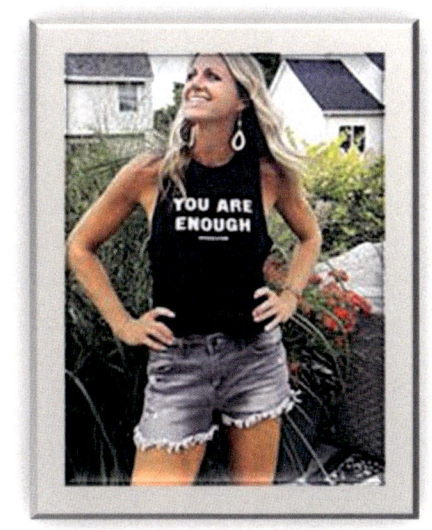

My name is Olivia Schmidt, born in Bettendorf, Iowa. I am a 41-year-old mother of two daughters who keep me busy and motivated to be the best version of myself in health and wellness. My love for fitness began in high school where I was a 4-sport athlete, leading to a Volleyball Scholarship to Minnesota State @ Mankato. There I graduated with a degree in Health Science. In 2003 I started participating in a Bootcamp program which lead to a passion for coaching and programming. I became a Bootcamp director and received my Level 1 CrossFit Certification. 8 years later I decided to take an incredible leap and start my own Bootcamp gym, Visionary Bootcamp. Each day I program a new challenging workout for my members. I currently have over 1000 workouts and have created multiple wellness challenges. I enjoy coaching individuals to reach their fitness goals. I hope by creating this book I can help you too!!! Coach Olivia/ Owner of Visionary Bootcamp

Table of Contents

Reference Key
Page 8-9

365 What's YOUR Vision Workouts
Pages 10-105

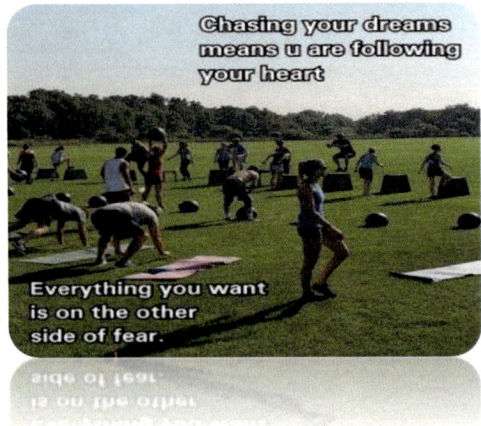

What's YOUR Vision Healthy 5 Week Challenge Page 106

Before and After Results Page 107

Week 1 Page 108

Week 2 Page 109

Week 3 Page 110

Week 4 Page 111

Week 5 Page 112

Weekly Notes and Score Sheet Page 113

Conclusion Page 114

Advice from the Author Page 115-117

FINALE Page 118

REFERENCE KEY

Refer to this key for some definitions of movements and definition of abbreviations.

Bf sit ups = butterfly sit ups. Ab mat behind your back, feet together in front. Touch the floor behind, swing arms up, and touch your feet in front.

SDLHP = Sumo deadlift to high pull. Can be used with a Kettle Bell or Barbell. With a straight back and strong shoulder blades, lower yourself down as low as you can without bending your upper or lower back. Tap on the floor raise up, as it crosses your hips arms shoot out, raise to your chin, right back down to the ground.

Hang Cleans = starting with weight at your hips, drive open hips and jump the weight to your shoulders like you are zipping up your coat.

Push press = Standing position, hold kettlebell or barbell on shoulders, dip with those legs and drive weight to overhead position back by your ears. Full extension of your arms.

Mountain Climbers = In a plank position, drive knees up as close to elbows as possible and alternate legs quickly on each side.

TTB = Toes to Bar. With your gymnastic kip lean back look at the bar, knees up and quick kick to bar. This is core so if you do not have a rig, modify it to a core movement.

PU = pullups. Gymnastic kip, head forward, feet back, as your feet whip forward, pull up, chin above the bar, push away up top.

GTO = Ground to overhead is with a plate or a bar. Chest shoulder back, touch the plate on the ground, flip at your chest and press overhead, plate parallel to the ceiling.

Swing = Kettlebell or an object. Load the hamstrings, knees slightly bent, hike the object back between your legs, pop those hips and extend the kettle bell all the way overhead, full extension of your arms. If it is a Russian swing, stop your swing at your chest.

Lunges = Big step forward, shin vertical lightly tapping the back knee on the ground.

Reverse Lunges = Big step backwards where shin is vertical, lightly tapping back knee on the ground.
Side Lunges= Both toes pointed forward, big step out to the side, where opposite leg is fully extended, accelerate back to starting point.
DU = Double under with a jump rope. Shoulders relax, elbows in, nice, and relaxed with your shoulders. Find the rhythm where the rope travels two times under each jump.

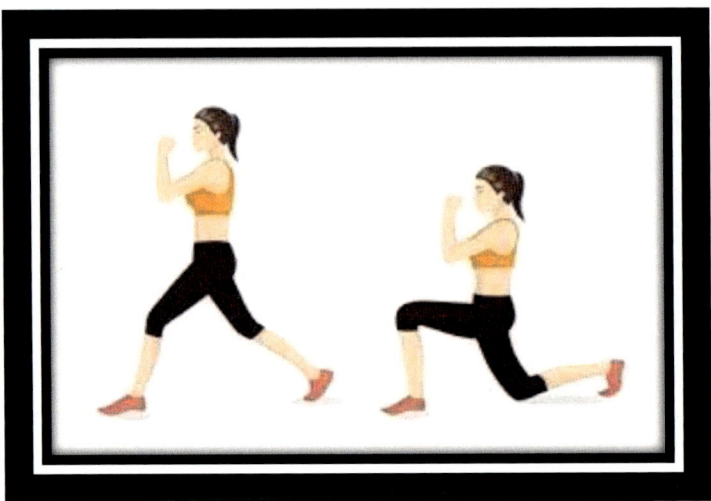

365 Bootcamp Workouts

1.) 7 rounds
100 m sprints
10 Pullups
10 Pushups
50 t climbers

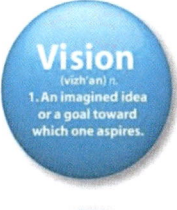

2.) 1000 m row
50 ball slams
20-2
Kb cleans
Overhead plate walking lunges
Squat thrust plate jumps
1000 m row
50 all slams

3.) 1 min plank
2 rounds
15 Sprints
15 Pullups mod pushups
15 Air squats
15 Kb swings
15 Setups
15 Burpees

4.) 10 rounds
10 Alt Kb snatch
10 box overs
10 Bf sit-ups
Every 2 min
30 du or 90 singles

5.) 25 min AMRAP
250 m row
15 kb swings 45/25
10 toes to bar
15 broad jumps
10 V twist (each side) 20/15

6.) 3,6,9,12,15,18,21
Russian swings 55/45
Burpee box jumps
Ring rows

7.) 100 wall balls
75 KB Cleans 45/25
100 Butterfly Sit ups
200 m run after each set

8.) 30 min wod
45 sec 15 sec rest
Min 1 box jumps
Min 2 hand release 1/2 burpees
Min 3 goblet squats

9.) 10 min AMRAP
100 m sprints
20 m seesaw press 45/25
1 min rest
25-20-15
Kb deadlifts 70/55
Kb pushups (2 kb)
BF sit ups
By out 100 walking lunges

10.) 5 rounds
500 m row
20 wall balls 24/14
12 bb strict press 65/45
1 min plank

11.) 4 rounds
800 m
30 air squats
20 broad jumps
10 kb clean and press. 45/25
Cash out 100 4 count flutter kicks

12.) 6 rounds
50 du
25 box overs
25 ground to overheads
25 straight leg sit ups

13.) Card deck
Plate thrusters
BF sit ups
Hr. 1/2 burpees
Bench jumps
Joker 1 30 broad jumps
Joker 2 60 m bear crawl

14.) 100 box jumps
100 Russian twist totals
100 air squats
100 kb swings 55/35
100 Cal row
Must complete exercise before moving on.

15.) 30 min AMRAP
400 m run
12 kb rdls 70/55
12 pull ups
5 hill sprints
20 bf sit ups
20 walking lunges

16.) 12-1
Burpee lateral ball jumps
Dead bugs
Kb bent over rows 55/35
Cardio of choice
30 du, 250 row, 200 m run after each set

17.) 21,18,15,9,6,3
Kb squat cleans
Burpees
Wall balls sit ups

18.) 6 rounds
1 min max reps
Wall balls
Wall balls sit ups
Burpees
Barbell bent over rows 75/45
1 min rest

19.) 28 min AMRAP
3,6,9,12..............
Toes to bar
Alt Kb snatches 45/25
Kb step ups
Start and Every 4 minutes 100 m shuttle sprints

20.) 4,8,12,16,20,24,28
Seesaw presses
Ball Slams
Then 100 du
28,24,20,16,12,8,4
Dead bugs 20/15
Wall Balls
Then 100 du

21.) 50 Air Squats
50 swings
By in
Then
7 rounds
10 deadlifts
10 squat thrust to plate jumps raises 15lb
100 m sprints
50 air squats
50 swings

22.) 4 rounds
10 ring rows
20 Pushups
30 Anchored sit ups
40 m 1 arm kb overhead 45/25
50 Bear Crawl
60 jump chins

23.) 50 mt climbers each
50 jump lunges each
50 straight leg sit-ups 35/20
50 barbell thrusters
50 kb straight leg sit ups

24.) 27 min AMRAP
30 Cal row
15 box jumps
15 ground to overhead
15 pull ups
1 min plank

25.) 30,25,20,15,10
Burpee bar touch
Alt kb snatch 45/25
After each set
20 ball slam 20/15
3 wall walks

26.) 8 rounds
60 m Sprints
10 Sumo Deadlift to high pull 70/45
1 min rest
Then
6 rounds
20 Air Squats
10 renegade rows 45/25
Then
4 rounds
20 lateral ball jumps
100 m sprints
2 rounds
50 Russian twist
59 flutter kicks

27.) 100 m farmers carry 70/55
100 m burpee broad jumps
Then
20-15-10-15-20
Pushups
Kb step ups 45/25
Box dips
Then
100m farmers carry
100 m burpee broad jumps

28.) 4 rounds
40 du
25 wall balls 20/15
30 du
25 kb swings 55/35
20 du
25 anchored sit-ups
10 du

29.) 5 rounds
50 m farmers carry 70/55
50 m walking lunges
Then
5 rounds
12 hr. 1/2 burpees
12 1 kb push press 45/25
12 kb straight leg sit-ups

30.) 35,25,15,25,35
Kb swings 55/35
2 rounds after each set
12 goblet squats 55/35
12 Barbell bent over
250 m row

31.) 100 du or 300 singles
60 ground to overhead 45/25
50 overhead plate walking lunges
40 bf sit ups
50 du
40 straight leg sit-ups
50 barbell push press 65/45
60 ground to overhead 45/25
100 du or 300 singles

32.) Death by 20
100 mt climber
4 rounds
24 Pullups
24 Box jumps
40m Bear crawl
Then
100 mt climber

33.) 5 rounds
1 min each exercise
Thrusters 75/55
Bear Crawl
Deadlifts
Dead bugs
Jump chins

34.) 4 rounds
500 m row
25 burpees
25 toes to bar
25 kb swings 55/35

35.) 50 dead bugs
Then
8 rounds
10 air squats
10 Kb swings
10 Burpees
10 air squats
10 kb swings
Then
50 dead bugs

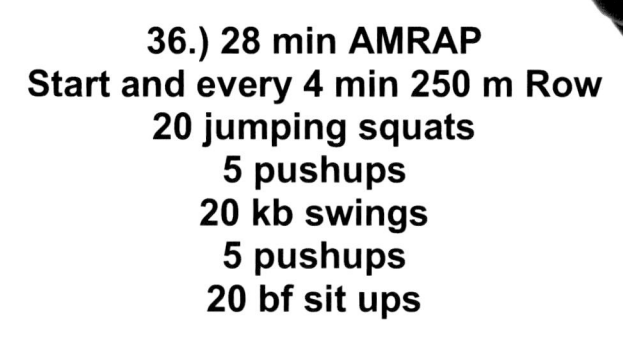

36.) 28 min AMRAP
Start and every 4 min 250 m Row
20 jumping squats
5 pushups
20 kb swings
5 pushups
20 bf sit ups

37.) 4 rounds
8 burpee bar jumps
25 barbell push press
8 burpees bar jump
20 ring rows
8 burpee bar

38.) 50-40-30-20-10
Kb stationary lunges 55/35
Box overs
30 du /90 singles after each set
Then
10-20-30-40-50
Kb swings
Anchored sit ups
30 du and 90 singles after each set

39.) 5 rounds

400m run
20 Kb snatch 45/25
20 v twist
200 m med ball rum
20 ball slams

40.) 2 rounds
500 m row
50 air squats
Then
2 rounds
500 m row
50 plate ground to overheads 45/25
Then
2 rounds
50 du
50 reverse stationary lunges
Then
2 rounds
50 du
50 lateral ball jumps (med ball)

41.) 10 min AMRAP
100 m sprints
20 m overhead plate walking lunges 45/25
15 ground to overheads 45/25
1-minute rest
4 rounds
20 sdlhp 55/45
20 sit up to plate raises 15 lb.
50 du or 150 singles

42.) 6 rounds
20 calorie row
After each row
2 rounds
20 Air Squats
10 barbell push press 85/55
10 anchored sit ups

43.) 21-15-9-15-21

Renegade Rows
Ball slams
Hr. 1/2 burpees
30 Russian twist after each set

44.) 2 rounds
500 m row
50 box jumps
50 1 arm kb push press 45/25
25 Cal bike
50 bf sit ups
50 kb swings 55/35

45.) 6 rounds
15 barbell bent over rows 75/55
30 Cal row
15 goblet squats 55/35
Beginning, after round 3, and end
50 bf sit ups(150total)

46.) 30 min AMRAP
25,20,15,10,5,10,15,20,25......
Burpee bar touch
Alt kb snatch 45/25
After each set
20 ball slam 20/15
3 wall walks

47.) 100 wall balls 20/14
80 kb swings 55/35
60 box jumps
40 pull ups
20 m bear crawl

48.) 5 rounds
1 min Sdlhp 75/55
1 min anchored sit ups
2 min bike
1 min walking lunges
1 min rest

49.) 7 rounds

12 Barbell strict press 30 du or 60

12 Med ball squat cleans
30 du
12 V twist

50.) 50,40,30,20,10
Cal row
After each row
16 Burpees
16 kb step up 45/35
16 dead bugs

51.) 75 du by in or 150
Then
5,10,15,20,25,30
Double kb squats 45/25
With 2 rounds after each set
5 pullups
5 pushups

52.) 10 rounds
10 push press 75/55
10 box overs
10 bf sit ups
Every other round 14 Cal bike or 2 min cardio
After rounds 2,4,6,8,10

53.) 30 min AMRAP
3,6,9,12,15,18,21
Burpee plate jumps 45/25
Kb swings 55/35
Overhead plate walking lunges 45/25
Kb windmills 35/25

54.) 3 rounds
1000 m row
25 wall balls
25 bent over rows 75/55
25 lateral ball jumps

55.) 7 rounds
20 m Seesaw presses 45/25
10 double kb step up 45/25
100 m sprints
10 Toes to bar

56.) 4 rounds
40 du
25 hr. 1/2 burpees
30 du
25 kb swings 55/35
20 du
25 anchored sit ups
10 du
25 air squats

57.) 5 rounds
16 Box overs
16 Ball slams
16 barbell strict press 65/45
4 burpees emom

58.) 30-20-10
Kb swings
Jumping lunges
Push press 75/55
10 Cal after each set
Then
10-20-30
Kb swings
Jumping lunges
Push press 75/55
15 Cal after each set

59.) 6 rounds
10 Alt kb thrusters 35/25
10 Toes to bar
50 Du or 150 singles
10 Kb Pushups

60.) 5 rounds
200 m sprints
40 ball slams
20 renegade rows 45/25

61.) Partner bike intervals
5 rounds each person
P1 10 Cal bike
P2 AMRAP kb swings 55/35
Then individually
21-15-9-15-21
Burpee bar touches
Pullups
50 du/150 after each set

62.) 30 min AMRAP
1000 m row
Remaining time
20 Bulgarian squats
20 bench dips
20 burpees
20 bf sit ups

63.) 30 min AMRAP
40 Cal bike
Start and at 15 min
20 Bulgarian squats
20 bench dips
20 alt swings 55/35
20 dead bugs

64.) 10,15,20,15,10,15,20
Wall balls 20/14
15 box jumps
15 kb deadlifts

65.) 2 rounds
750m row
40 kb reverse lunges 45/25
Then
2 rounds
500 m row
40 alt kb snatch 45/25
Then
2 rounds
250 row
40 Russian twist

66.) 5 rounds
1 min max reps
Barbell push press 75/55
Jump chins
Anchored sit ups
Squat thrust plate jumps
Ring rows
1 min rest

67.) 30 min AMRAP
Start and Every 5 min
20 Cal bike
40 du /120 singles
3,6,9,12,15,18,21.......
Box overs
Kb swings
Pushups

68.) 28 min AMRAP
10 pullups
20 ball slams
10 burpees
20 bf sit ups
Start and every 10 min (3 times total)
100 m farmers carry 70/55
20 m broad jumps

69.) 3 rounds
750 m row
15 swings 55/35
75 air squats
15 kb swings 55/35
25 barbell bent over rows 75/55
15 kb swings 55/35

70.) 75 anchored sit ups by in
Then
10 rounds
10 Kb thrusters 45/25
100 m sprints
10 box jumps

71.) 4 rounds
16 Cal bike
16 Renegade rows 45/25
20 m 2 kb front rack walking lunges 45/25
50 mt climbers

72.) 21-15-9-15-21
Barbell Thrusters 75/55
Dead bugs
Pushups
20m bear crawl after each set

73.) 10,20,30,20,10
Burpees
2 ROUNDS AFTER EACH SET
250 m row
10 barbell push press 75/55
10 ttb

74.) 3 rounds
2 min row
2 min kb swings
2 min Cal bike
2 min burpees
1 min rest

75.) 5 rounds
20 Wall balls
100 m sprints
15 pull ups
15 wall ball sit ups for height

76.) 2-20
Barbell strict press
75/55
Box jumps
Ball slams
30 du or 90 singles after ea
77.) 30 min AMRAP
30 kb cleans 45/25

30 Cal row
30 kb straight leg sit ups 45/25
60 walking lunges

78.) 50 Cal bike by in
Then
5 rounds
12 Ground to overheads
12 Toes to bar
24 Air Squats
12 Dumbbell front rack step ups 35/25

79.) Partner or individual
2 rounds
100 du or 300 singles
50 burpees
50 kb single arm push presses 45/25
50 bf sit ups
1000 m row

80.) 4 rounds
12 hr. 1/2 burpees
35 goblet squat 45/25
12 hr. 1/2 burpees
35 barbell sdlhp 75/55
12 hr. 1/2 burpees

81.) 50,40,30,20,10
Cal row
Kb swings 55/35
Bf sit ups
10 pull ups after each set

82.) 6 rounds
16 Wall balls
16 Renegade rows 45/25
20 Russian twist 24/14
40 du 120 singles

83.) 30 m AMRAP
16 Cal bike
20m Seesaw presses 45/25
30 Jump chins
20m single arm overhead walking lunges 45/25

84.) 10 rounds

10 ball slams

10 Sprints
10 Burpees
10 alt kb snatch 45/25

85.) 75 anchored sit ups
Then
50,40,30,20,10
Double under
Air Squats
1 min rest
5,10,15,20,25,30
Cal bike
Box jumps
Then
75 anchored sit ups

86.) 28 min AMRAP
Every min 4 burpees
10 toes to bar
20 box jumps

87.) 4 rounds
500 m row
25 alt dumbbell thrusters 35/20
50 du or 150 singles
1 min plank

88.) 50 kb swings 55/35
50 bf sit ups
50 kb reverse stationary lunges 55/35
50 pullups
50 kb reverse stationary lunges 55/35
50 bf sit ups
50 kb swings

89.) 30-20-10-20-30
Kb swings 55/35
Kb reverse lunges 55/35
400m run

90.) 2,4,6,8,10,12,14,16,18,20
Cal bike 0r interval running
Squat thrust to plate jumps
Kb sdlhp 70/55

91.) 1000 m row
75 air squats
50 kb step ups 45/25
50 bf sit ups
50 pullups
50 bf sit-ups
50 kb step ups
75 air squats
1000 m row

92.) 20, 30, 40, 30, 20 wall balls
Then
2 rounds After Each Set of wall balls
10 box overs
10 burpees
10 kb swings

93.) 3,6,9,12,15,21,24
Burpee bar jumps
After each set of burpees
12 barbell bent over row total 75/55
12 Box overs

94.) 3 rounds
30 kb swings
750 m row
30 bb push press 75/55
30 bb back rack forward stationary lunges 75/55

95.) 60 m bear crawl
Then
8 rounds
30 du or 90 singles
15 wall balls
10 pushups
Then
60 Russian twist 20/14

96.) 11 rounds
11 Hr. 1/2 burpees
11 Pullups
11 kb seesaw press
11 anchored sit ups with plate

97.) 20-2 (20,18,16,14,12,10,8,6,4,2)
Cal row
Kb swings
Box overs
Barbell strict 70/55

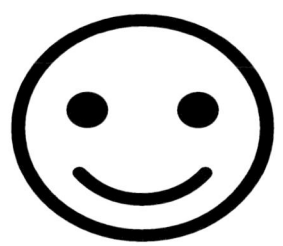

98.) 2 rounds
50 bf sit ups
20 burpees
50 air squats
20 burpees
50 Russian swings 55/35
20 burpees

99.) 750 m row
Then
4 rounds
20 kb snatches 45/25
20 kb reverse lunges
Then
750 m row
Then
4 rounds
20 med ball squat cleans 20/14
20 lateral ball jumps
Then
750 m row

100.) 5 rounds
30 Box overs
30 barbell push press 75/55
5 wall walks
400 m run
Each round decrease by 5

101.) 30 min AMRAP
Every 3 min
9 Cal bike or 200 m run
12 renegade rows 45/25
12 Kb push ups
12 Toes to bar
20 m broad jumps

102.) 100,80,60,40,20
ball slams
Du
After each set
15 Bench dips
20 Ground to overhead
25 jump chins
100 m sprints

103.) 100 anchored sit ups
4 rounds
500 m row
15 barbell sdlhp 75/55
15 burpee side jumps
15 kb swings 55/35
3 min plank

104.) 5 rounds
20m overhead walking lunges 45/25
20 Cal bike
20 box overs (if doing step ups add 25lb kb)
Then
100 4 CT flutter kicks

105.) 25-20-15-10-5
Barbell thrusters 75/55
10 burpee bar jumps
Toes to bar
10 burpee bar jumps

106.) Tabata
2 rounds thru whole thing (32 min wod)
4 rounds each exercise
40 sec on 20 sec off
Burpee plate jumps
Step up (chair, bench etc.) add kb ball etc.
Jump squats or goblet squats
Bf sit ups

107.) 30 min AMRAP
2 rounds
5 min
Bike, run, row, or sprint
1 min rest
5 min AMRAP
10 plank hip touches
10 lateral toe touches
10 Left knee right elbow alt
10 Squat thrust feet out in and stand
1 min rest
Last 10 min
2 min
Jumping jack low touches

108.) 4 rounds
20 Sdlhp kb/db. object
20 mt climbers
20 Straight leg to object/plate press oh
20 mt climbers
20 Lateral lunges total
20 mt climbers
Box jumps / object jumps
20mt climbers

109.) 50 1 arm push press kb db. object
50 kb goblet squats kb db.
50 1 arm bent over rows kb db. etc.
50 Russian twist total
5 min cardio (bike, row, run, jump. rope)
50 Russian twist total
50 1 arm bent over rows
50 goblet squats kb db.
50 1 arm push press kb / db.
(Ex. Of weight to press a handbag with canned goods, books in it, milk jug filled with water)
Switch as needed on all movement

110.) 6 rounds
1 min Bulgarian squats
1 min bf sit ups
1 min big lateral jumps toes touches
1 min hr. pushups
200 m run

111.) 21-15-9-15-21
Med ball squat cleans
Lateral ball jumps
Dead bugs
Hr. 1/2 burpees

112.) 10 rounds
After rounds, 2,4,6,8,10
400 m run or 2 min cardio
10 slam ball (if use med ball or basketball catch on bounce)
10 Bench dips
10 Bulgarian squats
. 30 sec plank

113.) 5 rounds
20 burpees
25 kb swings
30 walking lunges
35 parallel squats to knee to opposite elbow (leg core movement)

114.) 50,40,30,20,10
Box jumps
Du or (triple single)
Alt Russian swing kb or
25,20,15,10,5
Box (chair, bench) pushups to knee raise
Then
40 plank on hands leg raises

115.) 20,18,16,14,12,10,8,6,4,2
Clean to press kb/db. switch hands a n
Overhead squat kb/db. switch hands
Squat thrust kb jump
20 m bear crawl after each round or 50 mt climbers

116.) 2 rounds
thru everything
In a 7 min window
800m run, 1000 m row, 50 Cal bike
Home style wall balls
1 min rest
In a 5 min window
75 bf sit ups
Kb/object bent over rows remaining of time
1 min rest
In a 3 min window
50 high knees
50 jumping jacks clap behind
Forward plank remaining time
1 min rest

117.) CARD DECK WOD Flip each card
Hearts air squats
Diamonds inchworm push ups
Spades burpee deadlift kb/db
Clubs weighted step up kb/db
Joker 1 50 lateral ski jumps
Joker 2 50 alt v ups

118.) 350 walking lunges(stationary)total
Start and Every 4 min
10 hr. 1/2 burpees
10 shoulder tape from pushup

119.) 5 min cardio run /row/ bike
60 box jumps
4 min cardio
50 1 arm push press kb/db./object
3 min cardio

120.) 30 min AMRAP
20 Side squats
15 bench dips
20 shoulder taps
20 alt kb snatch
Every

121.) 30 min AMRAP
20 shuffle squats
20 alt kb snatch kb/db./object
20 bench dips
20 shoulder taps
Every 5 min 10 split thrust to tuck jump

122.) 100 du
90 kb swings
80 leg crunches on forearms
70 reverse lunge knees up
60 Russian twist
50 lateral object jumps
40 burpees
30 sec plank
20 pushups
10 rollbacks

123.) 5 rounds
1 min max reps
Weighted step ups with object
1 arm thrusters kb db. object
1 min cardio (bike, row, ropes, bear crawl)
Mt climbers
Sdlhp kb/db object

124.) 7 rounds
10 Lateral lunge alt toe touch
10 Floor press 1 kb/db
200 m run/or 1 min row/ bike
10 1 arm devils' press
10 dead bugs
200 m run or 1 min row/bike

125.) 100 burpees

Start and every 4 min 200 m run

20 kb swings
Wod is complete when 100 burpees are reached

126.) 5 rounds
20 Stationary lunge w/ball and twist
20 Med ball squat clean to press
400 m run
20 box jumps

127.) 10 rounds
30 Du 90 single or 30 high knees
8 Box pushups
8 Squat thrust mt climber to plate jump
20 m bear crawl (10 m forward, 10 m backwards)
After round 5 and 10 800m run

128.) 4 rounds
2 min window
30 Ground to overhead
Jump squats rest of time
5k run

129.) 25-20-15-20-25
Wall balls (show home wall balls to ceiling)
Bent over rows kb/db each side (50,40, 20.
Plank rolls total
(2 min cardio after each round)

130.) 800 m run (4 m cardio)
80 walking lunges
40 burpees lateral object jump
500 m run (3 min cardio)
60 walking lunges
30 burpee lateral object jump
300 m run (2 min cardio)

131.) 5 rounds
1 min max reps each exercise
1 min alt devils press kb
1 min jump rope or high knees
1 min dead bugs
1 min lateral ski jumps
1 min swing lunges (reverse to forward)

132.) 21,18,15,12,9,6,3
Squat jacks
Pushup climbs
Tiger kicks
Kb swings

133.) 3 rounds
30 Same leg weighted step ups w knee raise
(stay on each leg for 5 reps)
20 du /60 singles or 20 HK
30 weighted Straight Leg Sit up to side to side
20 Du/60 singles or 20 HK
30 push press kb/db and 20 du

134.) 4 rounds total
20 Sdlhp
10 Lateral ball jumps
10 hr. 1/2 burpees
20 Bulgarian squats
10 Lateral ball jumps
10 Hr. 1/2 burpees
20 Weighted bench dips
10 lateral ball jumps
10 hr. 1/2 burpees

135.) 105 total
Single arm thrusters
Every 15 reps
400 m run or 2 min cardio
15 box jumps
15 tiger kicks

136.) 800 m run or 4 min cardio

75 air squats
50 Kb swings
800m run 4 min cardio
75 air squats
50 kb swings

137.) 3 rounds
1 min each exercise
Bicycle crunches
Alt v ups
5 rounds
20 Jumps lunges stay on (same leg 5 reps)
20 Ground to overhead

138.) 2 times through everything (30 min wod)
4 min window
40 Squat thrust to Deadlifts
Du or singles jumping jacks remaining time
1 min rest
4 min window
40 Straight leg sit ups to press (plate object)
Raised quick toe taps remaining time
1 min rest

139.) 5 rounds
1 min max reps
Box overs mod step up (box, bench)
Alt kb/ db snatch
Lateral lunges (same leg 5 reps)
Russian twist
Broad jumps

140.) 2 mile run or 16 min cardio total
Every 2 min 20 shuffle squats
Ball slams

141.) 3 rounds
1 min high knees
1 min lateral ski jumps
1 min wall squat hold
Then
25,20,15,10,5
Weighted step ups
Alt kb Russian SWINGS
Hr. 1/2 burpees
400 m run or (2 min cardio)

142.) 30 min
Odd min 12 burpees rest remaining min
Even min cardio, row, run, bike, stairs, brisk walk
Then
40 straight leg sit up toe tap

143.) 5 rounds
400 m run
20 m walking lunges
30 mt climbers
20 broad jumps

144.) 2 rounds
800 m run (4 min cardio)
20 wall balls
20 kb swings
400 m run (2 min cardio)
20 wall balls
20 kb swings
200 m run (1 min cardio)
20 wall balls
20 kb swings
Then
3 min cash out
Forward side to side plank

145.) 75 anchored sit ups
Then
50,40,30,20,10
Cal bike
Weighted Walking lunges kb at chest 45/25
Russian twist with bicycle legs 20/15

146.) 6 rounds
1 min max each exercise
Weighted step ups to knee raises (same leg 5 reps) 35/25
Hr. 1/2 burpees
Barbell push presses
Plank up downs (hands to forearms etc.)
1 min rest

147.) 30 min AMRAP
1-mile run (8 min cardio)
Remaining time
16 renegade rows
5 pullups
16 bench dips
5 pullups
16 ball slams
5 pullups

148.) 30-20-10
Kb sdlhp 75/45
Box jumps
500 m row or 2 min cardio after
Then
10,20,30
1 arm db devils press 35/20
Box jumps
500 m row or 2 min cardio after each set
Cash out
50 scissor kicks
50 heel touches

149.) 5,10,15,20,25,30
Goblet squats 45/25
With 2 rounds after each set
10 ttb
30 du or 90 singles
200 m run
(12 rounds total)

150.) 3 rounds

200 m run
40 ball slams
200 m run
40 anchored sit ups
200 m run
40 kb swings

151.) 5 rounds
10 single arm kb squat clean to press 45/25
20 burpees
30 bicycle crunches
40 du or 120 singles

152.) 100 Cal bike
Every 10 Cal
10 box jumps
20 jumping lunges
10 alt kb snatch

153.) 27 min AMRAP
16 wall balls 20/14
18 dead bugs 20/14
20 kb Seesaw press 45/25

Every 4 min 200 m med ball run

154.) 10 rounds
10 barbell push press 75/55
10 kb swings 55/35
200 m run
Then
50 alt shoulder taps in plank

155.) 5 rounds
40 m Overhead walking lunges
20 burpees
10 Toes to bars
35 du or 105 singles

156.) 2 rounds

thru everything (32 min wod)
In a 6 min window
800m run,
Ground to overhead 45/25
rest of minute
1 min rest
In a 5 min window
400 m run
Kb/ bent over rows 55/35
remaining of time
1 min rest
In a 4 min window
200 m run
Broad jumps rest of minute
1 min rest

157.) 6 min ab burner AMRAP
20 knee crunches
20 heel touches
20 scissor kicks
Then
350 walking lunges total
Start and Every 4 min
200 m run
10 med ball squat cleans
Wod is complete after 350 lunges

158.) 50,40,30,20,10
Box jumps
Du or (triple single)
Alt Russian swing
12 Cal bike after each set.

159.) 10 rounds
After rounds, 2,4,6,8,10
400 m run
10 ball slams
10 burpees
10 1 arm kb push press 45/25

160.) 1-mile run
21,15,9,15,21
Barbell push press 75/55
T stab push ups
Jumping squats
Then
1-mile run

161.) 3 rounds
1 min each exercise
High knees
Ski jumps
Jumping jacks
Then
5 rounds
10 squat thrust to curb jumps
20 ball slams
30 Russian twist
400 m run

162.) 5 rounds
25 Burpee bar touches
25 box overs
5 wall walks
400 m run
Each round decrease by 5
Round 2 20 reps. 4 walks
Round 3 15 reps, 3 wall walks
Round 4 10 reps, 2 wall walks
Round 5 5 reps, 1 wall walks

163.) 3,6,9,12,15,18,21
Calorie Bike
Renegade rows 45/25
With
15 wall balls after 20/14
30 Russian twist 20/14
After each set

164.) 2 rounds

800 m run

50 kb swings
Then
3 rounds
400 m run
30 barbell push press 75/55
50 reverse lunges

165.) 4 rounds
40 Double under or 120 singles
20 alt kb snatch 45/25
4 rounds
40 air squats
20 hr. 1/2 burpees
4 rounds
40 bicycle crunches
200 m run

166.) 100 m farmer carry 70/55 by in
30-20-15-20-30
Ball slams
Pullups
Straight Leg plate raise
500 m row after each set
100 m farmer carry by out

167.) 2 rounds
50 box jumps
50 walking lunges
50 kb swings 55/35
400 m run AFTER EACH EXERCISE
(6 runs total)

168.) 4 rounds

10 burpee box jumps
200 m run
20 single arm kb thrusters 45/25
200 m run
20 bf sit ups
200 m run

169.) 1000 m row
Then 5 rounds
10 kb swings 55/35
10 pullups
10 Bulgarian squats
Then 1000 m row
3 rounds
15 kb swings
15 pushups
15 Bulgarian squats
Then 1000 m row

170.) 5 rounds
1 min Sdlhp 75/55
1 min Russian twist 20/15
2 min bike
1 min overhead plate walking lunges 45/25
1 min du or singles
1 min rest

171.) 20-15-10
Ball slams 20/15
Bench dips
Barbell Push press 75/55
400m run BEFORE each set
Then
40 dead bugs 20/15
Then

20-15-10
Ball slams
Bench dips
Barbell push press
400 m run BEFORE each set

172.) 1-mile run
Then
10 rounds
10 barbell bent over rows 70/55
10 Squat thrust bar jumps
10 toes to bar

173.) 3 rounds

200 m run
75 du or 225 singles
50 bf sit ups
400 m
40 air squats 20/15
20 Barbell strict press 65/45
800 m run
40 box overs

174.) 21-15-9-15-21
Weighted step ups
Bench dips
Single arm strict press
After each set
4 50 m shuttle sprints or 50 high knees
1 min plank

175.) 800 m run (4 m cardio)
80 walking lunges

40 med ball squat cleans
500 m run (3 min cardio)
60 walking lunges
30 med ball squat cleans
300 m run (2 min cardio)
40 walking lunges
20 med ball squat cleans
100 m run (1 min cardio)
20 walking lunges
10 burpee lateral object jump

176.)3 rounds
1 min electric chair therapy 20/15
1 min plank up downs
5 rounds
20 Rotational twist reverse lunges 20/15
100 m slam ball sprint
20 burpees
100 slam ball sprints (mod to step up)
20 toe touches with slam ball

177.)4 rounds

2 min window
25 Ground to overhead 45/25
Side ski jumps remaining time
2 min window
10 T stab push ups
Russian 1 arm swing 45/25 remaining time
2 min window
Du or singles max reps

178.)10 rounds
20 mt climbers

200 m run
10 kb single arm push press
10 Straight leg sit ups to plate raises
10 lateral same leg lunges (stay for 5 reps)

179.) 20,30,40,30,20
Box jumps
Ball slams
Then
3 rounds
30 Goblet squats (20/15)
400m run
30 Russian twist

180.) 120 wall balls
Start and ever 4 min
200 m run
10 hr. 1/2 burpees
Wod is complete when 120 wall balls are reached

181.) Core burner
3 rounds
20 bicycle crunches
20 Heel touches
20 Alt v ups
Then
2 rounds
800 m run
60 walking lunges
20 kb swings 55/35
10 pushups
400 m run

182.) 6 rounds
18 1 arm Bent over rows
18 Ball slams
40 Du or 120 singles
18 Squat thrust curb jump
Then

183.) 30 min AMRAP
10 Sdlhp 55/35
15 Bench dips
20 Plate sit ups
400 m run
Start and at 15 min mark
100 mt climbers
Every time u rest 20 high knees

184.) 1-mile trail run
Then
8 rounds.
8 Med ball squat cleans
16 Lateral ball jumps
16 Wall ball sit ups. Then
3 min plank hold

185.) 30-20-10-20-30
Burpees
Air Squats
After each set
200 m run
1 min plank

186.) 100 du
90 kb swings
800 m run

70 knee crunches
60 ground to overhead
50 Russian twist each
400 m run
30 side ski jumps
200 m run
10 rollbacks

187.) 2 rounds
1 min wall therapy
1 min hip touches in plank position
Then
5 rounds
20 Goblet squats 55/35
16 Elevated push ups
14 Single arm push press
400 m run

188.) 30 min
Min 1 10 burpees
Min 2 alt Russian kb swings
Min 3 overhead plate walking lunges
Min 4 box jumps

189.) 2 rounds
25 box jumps
400 m run
25 kb deadlifts 55lb
200 m run
50 bf sit ups
200 m run
25 kb deadlifts 55 lb.
400 m run
25 box jumps

190.) 60,50,40,30,20,10
Du singles
100 m sprint
Then
30,25,20,15,10,5
Wall balls
Dead bugs
100 m sprint

191.) 100 air squats
Then 7 rounds
200 m run
20 kb swings
10 squat thrust to push up
Then 100 air squats

192.) 3 rounds
400 m run
30 jumping lunges
Then
3 rounds
50 du or 150 singles
30 straight leg sit ups
3 rounds
400 m run
30 single arm bent over rows 55/35
Then
4 min
Burpee curb jump burnout

193.) 30-20-10
Ball slams 20/15
Bench dips
Then
1-mile run
75 Russian twist
Then
10-20-30
Slam ball thrusters 20/15
Lateral ball jumps tota

194.) 30 min AMRAP
Every 3 min
40 du /120 singles
3,6,9,12,15,18,21.......
Box overs
Stab pushups
Ground to overhead 45/25
Bf sit ups

195.) 2 rounds

1 min high knees
1 min knee crunches
1 min plank
Then
5 rounds
Squat jacks
Single arm push press
Burpee Broad jumps
400 m run

196.) 4 rounds
40 cross body mountain climbers
200 m run
30 kb swings 55/35
200 m run
20 kb stationary lunges 55/35

197.) 100,80,60,40,20
Du
Bicycle crunches
50,40,30,20,10
ball slams
Russian twist
After each set
400 m run

198.) 10 rounds
10 Overhead plate walking lunges
10 Sdlhp 70/55
10 Straight leg sit ups to plate raises
10 100 m med ball sprint

199.) 30 min AMRAP
1-mile run
40 broad jumps
Then remaining time
10 inchworm push ups
15 kb swings 55/35
20 Box jumps

200.) 800m run
15 Med ball squat cleans
15 Kb single arm bent over rows
15 Alt v ups
400m run

20 med ball squat cleans
20 kb single arm bent over rows
20 alt v ups
200m run
25 med ball squat cleans

201.) 4 rounds
40 Double under or 120 singles
20 ground to overhead 45/25
3 rounds
400 m run
20 hr. 1/2 burpees
2 rounds
40 alt Russian swings
200 m run

202.) 3 rounds
200 m run
40 med ball squat cleans
200 m run
40 dead bugs
200 m run

203.) 5 rounds
20 reverse lunges with kb press (stay on 1 leg for 5)
400 m run
20 squat thrust to deadlifts
1 min plank hold

204.) 4 rounds

2 min window
20 Ground to overhead
Jumping squats rest of time
2 min window
20 kb swings 55/35
Jump rope rest of time
2 min window
20 bf sit ups
Box jumps rest of time
205.) 6 rounds
12 bench dips
5 burpees
12 weighted Bulgarian squats
5 burpees
12 alt twist v ups
5 burpees
200 m run

206.) 800 m run
Then
100, 75, 50, 25
Air Squats
Mt climbers
After each set
400 m run
10 Broad jumps
10 Pushups
4 rounds
800 m run
After each run
2 rounds
10 Sdlhp
10 Box overs

207.) 5 rounds
15 wall balls
400 m run
15 wall balls
30 Russian twist
30 kb swings

208.) 150m farmer carry 70/55
800 m run by in
Then
30-20-15-20-30
Ball slams
Single arm bent over rows 45/35
Straight leg weighted ball sit ups
Then
150 m farmer carry
800 m run by out

209.) 5 rounds
1 min max each exercise
Weighted step ups same leg for 5 reps
Hr. 1/2 burpees
Du or singles
Plank up downs (hands to forearms etc.)
200 m run
1 min rest starts when last person comes in from run

210.) 25,20,15,10,5
Kb Deadlift to squat clean 45/35
Pushups
Dead bugs
After each set
30Du or 90singles
400 m run

211.) 2 rounds
1 min heel touch
1 min knee crunches
1 min bicycle crunch
Then
1-mile trail run
8 rounds
10 Kb swings
10 ball slams
10 Kb push press
1-mile trail run

212.) 4 rounds

20 burpee box jumps
20 single arm kb thrusters 75/55
Then
800 m run
50 anchored sit ups

213.) 3 rounds
200 m run
40 ground to overheads
200 m run
40 alt v ups
200 m run
40 swing lunges

214.) 40-30-20-10
Kb swings
With 2 rounds after each set
10 stab pushups
30 du or 90 singles
400 m run
(8 rounds total)

215.) 4 rounds
2 min Wall balls 20/15
1 min Russian bicycle twist 20/15
2 min Box jumps
1 min Bench dips
1 min rest
Cash out
800 cool down

216.) 8 rounds
2 hill sprints
50 mt climbers
10 side lunges
10 Sdlhp 55/35

217.) 2 rounds (32 min wod)

In a 6 min window
800m run,
Jump squats remaining time
1 min rest
In a 5 min window
400 m run
Bf sit ups remaining time
1 min rest
In a 4 min window

200 m run
Burpees remaining time
1 min rest

218.) 1000 m row
60 box jumps
500 m row
25 barbell push press 75/55
250 m row
25 barbell push press 75/25
500 m row
60 box jumps
1000 m row

219.) 10 rounds
10 wall balls 20/14
10 hr. 1/2 burpees
Then
800 m run
Then
3 rounds
20 goblet squats 55/35
200 m run

220.) 50,40,30,20,10
DU or triple singles
kb swings
BF sit ups
15 pull ups after each set

221.) 61 burpees by in
5 rounds years
4 ctb /pull ups
30 box jumps
400 m run
6 barbell thrusters 95/75
7 kb heavy swings 70/55

222.) 100 Cal on bike
Every 10 Cal
20 m walking lunges
10 db alt snatches 45/25
Then
100 Russian twist w slam ball 20/15
Workout is complete when you reach 100 calories.

223.) 30 min AMRAP
100 air squats and buy in
12 ground to overheads 45/25
12 pushups
12 broad jumps
Start and Every 4 min
200 m run
Cash out
40 dead bugs

224.) 100 bf sit up
Then
21,18,15,12,9,6,3
Kb swings 55/35
200m run
Barbell bent over rows 75/55
30 du or 90 singles

225.) 5 Rounds for Time
15 toes to bar
15 kb stationary lunges 45/25
400 m run or 500 m row
15 MB squat Cleans (20/14)

226.) 4 rounds

15 Cal bike
15 barbell strict press 95/65
After each set 2 rounds
10 kb swings 55/35
10 pushups

227.) 21-15-9-15-21
Alt. db snatch 45/25
Box overs
50 du or 150 singles
250 m row
25 dB Thrusters 45/20
25 Kb swings 55/35
25 anchored sit ups
400 m run
Round 2 20 reps
Round 3 15 reps
Round 4 10 reps
Round 5 5 reps

228.) 5 K run/ row

229.) 5 rounds
5 min AMRAP
10 ring rows

50 du or 150 singles
15 kb deadlift 70/55
Cal bike remainder of the time
1 min rest

230.) 20-2 (20,18,16,14,12,10,8,6,4,2)
Box jumps
Ground to overhead 45/25
Hr. pushups
2 hill sprints after each round

231.) 30 min AMRAP
10 burpee box jumps
400 m run
10 barbell push press
10 bf sit ups

232.) 5 rounds
12 wall balls
400 m run
12 box jumps
12 kb swings

233.) 800 m run
25-15-10-15-25
Renegade rows
Double KB front rack stationary lunges
Then
800 m run

234.) 100 Dumb bell snatches
Start and every 2 min 25 air squats
Then
4 rounds
400 m run/ 500 m row hard
1 min rest
Max effort

235.) 5 rounds
1 min max reps each exercise
1 min Cal bike
1 min KB SDLHP
1 min pullups
1 min burpee bar touches
1 min rest

236.) 2 rounds
80 du or 240 singles
50 alt Russian swings
60 du or 180 singles
50 box overs
40 du or 120 singles
50 ball slams
20 du or 60 singles
50 Russian twist

237.) 5 rounds
20 Ground to overheads
20 Goblet Squats
20 KB pushups
400 m run

238.) 7 rounds
250 m row
16 box jumps
14 kb deadlifts
10 burpee lateral jumps

239.) 3 rounds
800 m run
30 wall balls
20 toes to bar
30 straight leg sit ups

240.) Core burner buy in
3 rounds
1 min Russian twist 20/15
1 min alt v ups
1 min plank
(no rest between rounds)
Then
1 min rest
Then
3 rounds
20 Overhead plate reverse lunges 45/25
800 m run
20 Pull Ups

241.) 21-15-9-15-21
Cal bike
Barbell push press
After each set
50 du or 150 singles
50 m Farmers Carry

242.) 2 rounds
800m run
40 jumping lunges
20 Kb swings
10 pushups
Then 2 rounds
400 m run
20 jumping lunges
20 KB swings
10 pushups

243.) 24,20,16,12,8, 4
Hand Release Burpees
250 m row
Pullups
250 m row

244.) 5 rounds
20 medicine ball squat cleans
20 box jumps
20 dead bugs
400 m run

245.) 100 air squats
100 anchored sit ups
100 kb swings
100 reverse lunges
200 m run every 4 min

245.) 1-mile run
5 wall walks
Then
5 rounds
10 weighted steps up
10 bench dips
10 Alt snatches

246.) 5 rounds
20 Wall Balls
200 m Med ball run
15 Toes to bar
100 m run
10 Db single arm bent over rows

247.) 50,40,30,20,10
Cal bike
After each set
15 burpees
20 walking lunges

248.) 4 rounds
400 m run
With 3 rounds after each run of
10 Box overs
10 push press
20 Du or 60 singles

249.) 30 min AMRAP
800 m Run at start and 15 min mark
15 Goblet squats
15 swings
10 Kb pushups
10 pull ups

250.) 5 wall walks
800 m run
30-25-20-15-10-5
Wall balls
BF sit ups
Bench dips
Then
1200 m run

251.) 5 rounds
250 m sprints
15 deadlifts
Then 5 rounds
10 kb renegade rows
20 russian twist Then 800 m run

252.) 3 rounds
800 m run
50 Du or 150 singles
20 Side lunges
20 Barbell strict press

253.) 100 balls slams
90 kb swings
80 swings
70 mt climbers
60 sec plank
50 burpees
40 air squats
30 pushups
20 broad jumps
10 hill sprints

254.) 25 Cal bike
Then 3 rounds
16 KB SDLHP
16 pullups
25 Cal Bike

255.) 20-2
Thrusters
Box jumps
Dead bugs
200 m run

256.) 2 rounds
1 min wall therapy
30 sec plank
Then 8 rounds
200 m run
10 step ups
30 du or 90 singles
10 single arm devils press

257.) 3 rounds
400 m run
60 m Farmers Carry
60 m Walking lunges
Then 3 rounds
16 KB cleans
12 toes to bar

258.) 10 Rounds
10 Barbell Strict Press
200 m run
Then 1000 m row
Then 3 rounds
20 goblet squats
250 m row

259.) 5 rounds
1 min max reps each exercise
Burpees
Anchored sit ups
Cal Row
2 KB front squats
1 min rest

260.) 20-2
Overhead plate walking lunges
Plate jumps
10-1
Toes to bar
Hr. 1/2 burpees
After even rounds 400
After odd 30 sec plank

261.) 12 rounds
12 ground
12 box overs
12 Russian swings
Every 4 min 200 m run

262.) 3 rounds

3 min AMRAP
8 pullups
8 pushups
1 min rest
3 min AMRAP
8 kb squat cleans 45/25
10 bf sit ups
1 min rest
3 min AMRAP

30 du or 90 singles
50 Mt climbers

263.) 3 rounds
25 strict 65/45 press set down 3 burpees
400 m row
25 Wall balls set down 3 burpees
400 m row
40 m bear crawl

264.) 5 rounds
1 min each exercise
front rack kb lunges 45/25
Ring rows
Sdlhp
Bench jumps
Ball slams

265.) 5 hill sprints
50 step ups
5 hill sprints
50 jump chins
50 wall ball sit ups
5 hill sprints
50 goblet squats
5 hill sprints
50 m bear crawl
5 hill sprints

266.) 1 mile for time
21,18,15,12,9,6,3
Kb swings 55/35
Box overs 24/20
5 burpees after each set

267.) 10 rounds
10 toes to bar
10 kb swings 55/45
10 box overs
After round 2,4,6,8,10
40 du after each set

268.) 4 rounds
500 m row
20 kb stationary lunges 45/25
20 kb snatches 45/25
50 du or 150 singles
20 bf sit ups

269.) 10 rounds
2,4,6,8,10 50 du or 150 singles
2 rounds
10 pushups
15 swings
20 air squats

270.) 28 min AMRAP
400 m run
10 ring rows
15 kb deadlifts
20 ball slams
25 Russian twist

271.) Partner 1
4×200 rest
Partner 1
100 kb thrusters
Switch every 10
Partner 1
3 400
Rest
Partner 1
100 seesaw press
Switch ever 10
800 run together

272.) 40 sec on 20 min rest

2 min each exercise
4 rounds
Cal Row
Burpee rower jumps
Ground to overhead 45/25
Seesaw presses 45/25
Cash out 40 straight leg sit-ups

273.) 800 m by in
5 rounds
20 Wall balls
15 Ring rows
20 Straight leg sit ups
4 hill sprints

274.) 50 wall balls
50 rds.
50 jump chins
50 box jumps
50 push presses
50 burpees
50 bf sit ups
50 du
500 m run

275.) 3 rounds
800 m run
50 air squats
40 kb swings
30 ball slams
20 pull ups

276.) 5 wall walk by in
10-1
Renegade row
Front lunges
Wall ball sit ups
Lateral jumps each side
5 wall walks by out

277.) 4 rounds

500 m row
20 Kb snatches 45/25
30 Kb v twist total
30 Box jumps
20 m bear crawl

278.) 1-mile run
Then
6 rounds
21 wall balls
15 pushups
9 kb rollbacks
Then
1-mile run

279.) 5 rounds
200 m med ball run
15 Toes to bar
15 Suitcase deadlifts
4 hill sprints
15 hr. half Burpee

280.) 4 rounds
2 min max row
1 min max swings
1 min max box overs
1 min max bf sit ups
2 min max air squats
1 min rest

281.) 800 m run
40 clusters 75
40 toes to bar
100 du
60 wall balls
60 pull ups
60 power snatches 75
1000 m row

282.) 100 strict press

100 wall balls height
100 deadlifts
100 jump chins
2000 m run

283.) 7 min AMRAP
20 m Farmers carry
10 Bear crawl
10 Squat thrust Broad jumps
Then
4 rounds
20 kb step ups
20 ring rows
50 du Or 125 singles
50 Russian twist total

284.) 2 rounds
800 m run
40 wall balls
40 bf sit ups
Then
3 rounds
400 m run
15 kb clean to press 45/25
25 box jumps
Then
4 rounds
200 m run
15 ball slams

285.) 20-2
Box jumps
Goblet squats
Bench dips
200 m run after each set

286.) Partner wod or individual

2 rounds
1000 m row total
P1 250 m
P2 ground to overheads
60 kb cleans total
P1 10 kb cleans 55/35
P2 jumping lunges
60 squat thrust to ball jumps
P1 10 at a time
P2 side ball slams

287.) 30 min AMRAP
1-mile run
25 broad jumps
Then remaining time
20 pull ups
25 ground to overheads
200 m med ball carry
30 straight leg kb sit ups
5 wall walks

288.) 800 m run
500 m row
100 du or 300 singles
Then 2 rounds
50 air squats
3 wall walks
50 Russian swings
3 wall walks
50 lateral ball jumps
3 wall walks
Then
800 m run
500 m row
100 du

289.) 50,40,30,20,30,40,50
Du or triple singles
After each set
200 m run
10 burpees box jumps
10 kb squat cleans

290.) 2 rounds
70 du or
12 burpees
50 wall balls
12 burpees
30 bf sit ups
12 burpees
20 kb push presses 45/25
12 burpees

291.) 50 sit-ups
30 kb thrusters
20 pushups

292.) 1000 m row
25 kb snatches
25 reverse lunges
25 Russian twist
750 m row
20 kb snatch
20 reverse lunges
20 Russian tw

293.) 10 rounds
200 m run
10 seesaw press 45/25
10 Ball slams
10 bench jumps

294.) 21-15-9-15-21

Pullups
Hr. 1/2 burpees
Kb step ups
Bent over rows
Cash out
800 for time
30 ghd sit-ups

295.) 1 mile by in
4 rounds
20 wall balls
20 walking lunges total
20 bb Strict press 65/45
200 m med ball run

296.) 4 rounds
400 m run
25 goblet squats
25 box overs
25 Burpee bar touches

297.) 21,18,15,12,9,6,3
Cal row
Overhead plate walking lunges 45/25
Ground to overheads
Burpee plate jumps
Cash out 3 min plank

300.) 5 rounds
4 hill sprints
45 du or 90 singles
25 box jumps
15 kb clean to press 45/25

301.) 15 Wall balls
10 Pullups
5 Kb rollbacks
400 m run

302.) 4 min AMRAP

8 wall balls
8 Pullups
8 kb rollbacks
1 min rest
5 min AMRAP
10 wall balls
10 pullups
20 m broad jumps

1 min rest
6 min AMRAP
12 Wall balls
12 pull ups
20 m bear crawl
1 min rest
7 min AMRAP
14 wall balls
14 pullups
200 m run

303.) 4×400m run
1 min rest in between each run
Then
4 rounds
16 suitcase deadlifts 55/35
16 Bulgarian squats (no weight)
16 squat thrust to bar touches
16 Dead bugs 20/14
Then
4 ×200 med ball run
30 sec rest in between each run

304.) 20, 30, 40, 30, 20 box jumps
Then
2 rounds After Each Set of box jumps (10 times through)
10 Ball slams
10 kb swings 55/35
8 toes to bar

305.) 50 du or 100 singles

50 Cal row
50 jump chins
50 Bf sit ups
50 kb rdls 70/55
50 pushups
50 lateral ball jumps
50 calorie row
50 du or 100 singles
306.) 3 rounds
2 min
15 box overs
1/2 burpees rest
1 min rest
3 rounds
2 min
200 m run
Mt climbers rest
1 min rest
3 rounds
2 min
30 m bear crawl
Barbell bent over rows

307.) 100 m farmers carry 70/55 by in
8 rounds
12 Wall balls 24/20
12 Kb swings 55/35
20 Russian twist 20/15
1 mile by out

308.) 4 rounds
20 m front rack lunges
10 Kb cleans
Then 1 min plank
4 rounds
10 Pullups
10 Burpee broad jumps
1 min plank
4 rounds
10 Ball slams
10 dead bugs

309.) 28 min AMRAP
3,6,9,12,15,18,15,12,9......
Burpees
Kb push presses
Box overs
Start and every 4 min 7 pullups

310.) 20-2
Cal row
Ground to overheads
After 20,16,12,8,4
30 m walking lunges
3 hill sprints
Cash out 100 Russian twist

311.) Partner wod
2 rounds thru
60 cleans switch every 10 pc
P1 kb cleans 55/25
P2 straight leg sit ups
400 run together
60 pull-ups switch every 10 pull-ups
P1 Hr. pushups
P2 Lateral ball jumps
400 run together
60 ball slams switch. every 20
P1 Ball slams 20/15
P2 plank hold
400 together

312.) 10 rounds
(Choose your cardio), mix them up or stay with same one all 10 rounds
35 du or 105 singles/ or 200m run or 200m row
10 Wall balls
10 kb deadlifts 75/55
10 Russian twist each side 20/15

313.) 70,60,50,40 du
After each set
3 rounds
8 pushups
8 ttb
8 burpees

314.) 4 rounds
400 m run
20 kb snatches
15 ttb
50 4 CT flutter

315.) 50,40,30,20,10
Box jumps
After each set
2 rounds
10 barbell strict press 65/45
10 barbell front rack stationary lunges 65/45
10 burpees

316.) 3 rounds total
2 min max row
4 min AMRAP
12 kb swings 55/35
12 pushups
1 min rest
2 min max du
4 min AMRAP
12 Wall balls
12 bf sit ups
1 min rest

317.) 800 m run
70 m farmers carry
70/55
3 wall walks
200 run
60 ground to overhead
3 wall walks
200 m run
50 jump chins
3 wall walks
200 m run
40 sdlhp 70/55
3 wall walks 800 m run

318.) 6 rounds

100 m sprint (top of hill)
16 Kb step ups
30 Air Squats
100 m sprint
16 Kb 1 arm push press 45/25 Alt as needed
Wall sit ups for height

319.) 4 rounds
Partner I go u go
250 m row
50 du
Then
1-mile run
21-15-9
Pullups
Wall balls
Hr. 1/2 burpees

320.) 30 min AMRAP
400 m run
10 overhead plate walking lunges 45/25
10 Ring rows
10 bf sit ups
Each round increase by 5 reps after run

321.) Round 1
2 rounds
800m run
75 air squats
Round 2
2 rounds
400 m
50 box jumps
2 rounds
200 m run
50 alternating swings
2 rounds
3 hill sprints
50 bf sit ups

322.) 800 m run

50 du or 100 singles
50 Bf sit ups
50 box jumps
50 bb push press 65/45
200 m med ball run
50 burpees bar touches
50 ball slams
50 du or 100 singles
800 m run

323.) 16-2 decrease by 2 each set
Kb clean to press 45/25
Toes to bar
V twist each side 20/15
200 m run after each set
8 total runs

324.) 10 squat thrust to plate jumps
10 bench dips
400 m row
20 bench dips
20 squat ....
400 m row
30 bench dips
30 squat thrust plate jumps
200 m run
30 straight leg sit ups
30 wall balls
400 m row
20 Straight leg sit
20 wall balls
400 m row
10 straight leg sit ups

325.) 50 wall ball by in
4 rounds. each round increase reps by 10
400 m row
10 squat thrust plate jumps
10 kb sdlhp
10 plate raise sit ups

326.) 4 rounds
10 wall balls
10 lateral ball jumps
10 pushups
20 du or 80 singles jump ropes

327.) 3 rounds
20 m kb front rack walking lunges 45/25
30 jump chins
20 m kb seesaw presses
800 m run
Then
100 air squats by out
100 4 CT flutter kicks

328.) 6 rounds
3 sprints
75 mt climbers
20 box jumps
10 pushups
3 wall walks

329.) 10 rounds
6 pull ups
8 alt kb snatches 45/25
10 wall balls
After Rounds 1,3,5,7,9 400 m run
After Rounds 2,4,6,8,10
3 hill sprints

330.) 2 rounds
70 du or
12 burpees
50 wall balls
12 burpees
30 bf sit ups
12 burpees
20 kb push presses 45/25
12 burpees

331.) 5 rounds

1 min
Row
Burpee jumps
Ball slams
Setups
200 med ball run

332.) 800 m run
100 du or 300 singles
Then 2 rounds
50 air squats
3 wall walks
50 Russian swings 55/35
3 wall walks
50 Russian twist
3 wall walks
Then
800 m run
100 du or 300 singles

333.) 30 min AMRAP
1-mile run
50 burpee plate jumps
Remaining time
20 jump squats
20 kb push ups
20 pull ups

334.) 10,20,30,40,50
Wall balls
Lateral ball jumps
After each set
400 m run
40 m walking lunges
1 min plank

335.) 2 rounds
800 m run
20 bent over rows
20 broad jumps
400 m med ball run
50 ball slams

336.) 24,21,18,15,12,9,6,3
Kb swings
3 burpees
Box jumps
3 burpees

337.) 3 rounds
800 m run
50 air squats
40 bf sit ups
30 seesaw presses 45/25
20 pull ups

338.) 4 rounds
Bike 1 min
8 Push press
8 Walking lunges
5x200 sprints
4 rounds
10 Kb step ups
10 Ground to overheads
Jump ropes

339.) 200 m run
10 Pushups
10 Ball slams
10 Burpee lateral ball jumps
400 m run
20 Pushups
20 Ball slams
20 Burpees lateral ball jump jumps
800 m
30 Pushups
30 Ball slams
30 Burpee
1-mile run

340.) 5 rounds
500 m row
2 rounds
10 pullups
10 pushups

341.) Reps 24,18,12,18,24
Barbell push presses 65/45
Kb step up 45/25
Box dips
50 du or 150 singles after each set 5 total
Cash out
30 glute ham raises

342.) 4 min burpee plate jumps by in
Then 1000 m run
2 rounds
50 ball slams
50 walking lunges
25 hr. 1/2 burpees
1 min plank hold
Then 1000 m run

343.) 2 rounds
1 min row
1 min box overs
1 min wall walks
1 min kb snatches
1 min rest
2 rounds
2 min row
2 min box overs
2 min wall walks
2 min kb snatches
1 min rest

344.) 5 min AMRAP
100 m shuttle sprints
20 m squat thrust to broad jumps
Then
21,18,15,9,6,3
Kb thrusters 45/25
Toes to bar
Kb swings 55/35
30 du or 90 singles after each set

345.) 10 rounds

10 Wall balls
10 Seesaw presses
10 bf sit ups
Emom 20 mt climbers

346.) 8 min AMRAP
8 Ring rows
8 Plate overhead walking lunges 45/25
8 Burpee box jumps
1 min rest
10 min AMRAP
10 ring rows
10 plate overhead walking lunges
10 burpee box jumps
10 Russian twist
1 min rest
12 min AMRAP
12 ring rows
12 overhead walking lunges
12 burpee box jumps
12 Russian twist

347.) 12 min AMRAP
8 ring rows
10 kb swings
10 plate lunges
1 min bike

348.) 4 rounds
500 Row
3 rounds
5 pushups
10 Ground to overhead
10 barbell bent over rows

349.) 3 rounds
800 m row
30 alternating swings 55/35
30 air squats
30 pullups
30 V twist 20/15

350.) 30-20-10-20-30
Box jumps
Kb sdlhp 55/35
200m run after each set
20-15-10-15-20
Strict press 55/35
Straight Leg sit ups
200 m run after each set

351.) 5 rounds
50 du 150 singles
12 Burpees
12 toes to bar
20 Reverse lunges
Cash out
2 rounds
1 min wall therapy
1 min plank

352.) 3 rounds
50 wall balls
30 kb alt snatches 45/25
1 min plank
Cash out

353.) 20 m bear crawl
Then
25,20,15,10
Deadlift 70/55
Burpee kb jumps
Then
40 m bear crawl
Then
25,20,15,10
Ball slams
Kb step up
Then
60 m bear crawl

354.) 75 bf sit ups by in
Then
10 rounds
7 Kb squat cleans 45/25
7 Pullups

355.) 7 rounds
60 m sprints
10 hr. 1/2 burpees
1 min rest
Then 5 rounds
10 push press 65/45
10 bb front rack stationary lunges
1 min rest
Then 3 rounds
12 pushups
20 alt v ups

356.) 21-15-9-15-21
Cal row
Box overs
Ground to overheads 45/25
Straight leg sit ups to plate raises 45/25

357.) 22 min AMRAP
20 bench dips
50 Jump chins
20 Toes to ring
50 kb swings
E2mom 10 jump squats

358.) 5 rounds
25 wall balls
20 lateral ball jumps
15 ring rows
10 burpees
100 m sprints

359.) 6 rounds
250 m row
20 m seesaw press 45/20
20 bf sit ups
Then
2 rounds
50 ball slams
1 min plank

360.) 2 rounds

50 du or 150 singles
50 Bf sit ups
40 du or 120 singles
50 bb bent over rows 55/75
30 du or 90 singles
50 ball slams 20/15
20 du or 150 singles
50 goblet squats (slam ball)
10 du or 30 singles

361.) 10 min AMRAP
10 Wall balls
10 sprints
2 min rest
5 rounds
10 Kb cleans to press 45/25
50 mt climbers

362.) 3 rounds
1000 m row
25 pullups
25 suitcase deadlift 45/25 (2 kb)
25 Bf sit ups
1 min electric chair 25/15

363.) 30 burpee bar touch
100 anchor sit ups
100 lateral ball jumps
30 hr. 1/2 burpees
100 Russian twist
100 stationary lunges
30 squat thrust

364.) 2 rounds

750 m row
75 air squats
Then
2 rounds
500 m row
50 bf sit ups
Then
2 rounds
250 row
50 barbell push press 55/35

365.) 4×250
30 sec rest
4 rounds
10 air squats
10 pushups
10 sit ups
4x 5 burpees 30 sec rest

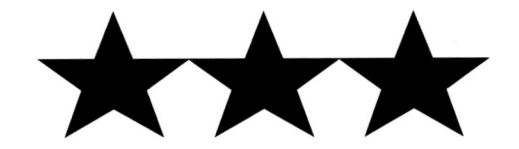

★★★

HEALTHY LIFESTYLE 5 WEEK DAILY CHALLENGE

This section of the book is a 5-week Healthy Lifestyle Challenge. I have written a daily challenge plus bonus challenge for every day of the week for 5 weeks. Your goal is to try and complete as many daily challenges as you can.

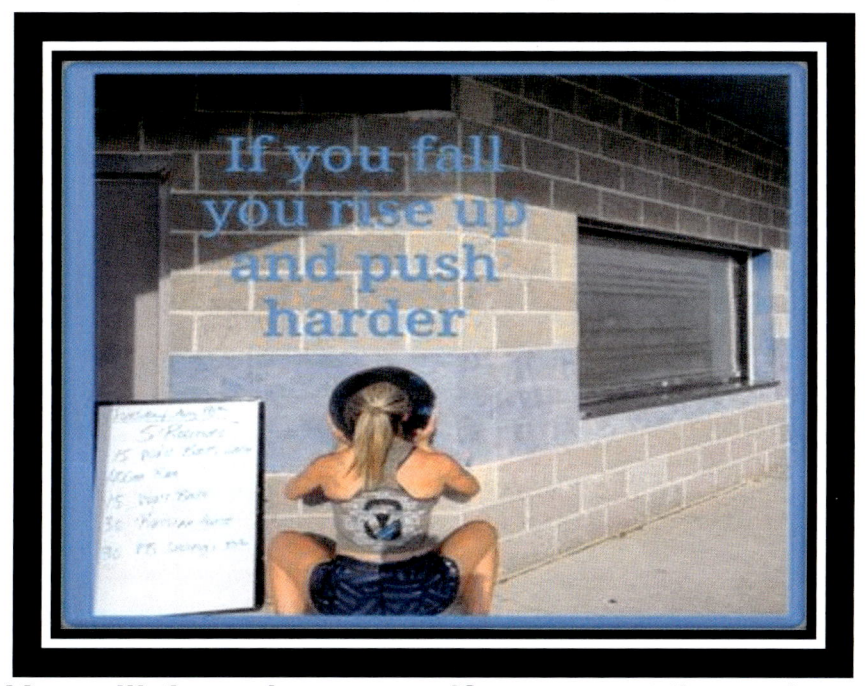

You will then give yourself a score at the end of the week on the points page. This is your accountability score. These challenges vary from fitness, nutrition, to self-evaluation and self-goals. Do the best you can.

You got this!

BEFORE AND AFTER RESULTS PAGE

This is optional. You can take a picture and do measurements before you commit to this challenge and once you complete it! Results are Motivation!

BEFORE	AFTER
Hips	Hips
Stomach	Stomach
Right Thigh	Right Thigh
Left Thigh	Left Thigh
Right Bicep	Right Bicep
Left Bicep	Left Bicep

Before | **After**

WEEK 1

Monday
Record a measurable exercise and nutritional goal for yourself during this challenge. Weigh yourself, record the data. Also, recommend taking side, back, and front pictures of yourself.

Tuesday
150 total burpees for the day.

Wednesday
Guys consume 150 plus grams of protein. Ladies consume 120 grams of protein.

Thursday
Drink 8 plus cups of water!

Friday
200 Walking lunges, modify to stationary if needed

Saturday
30 min of Cardio at one time. Example: Run, walk, bike, hike,

Bonus weekly point
Accumulate 5 extra running miles. If you are not able to run, try brisk walk and modify distance if needed, but challenge yourself!

WEEK 2

Monday
Find a healthy crock pot recipe and prepare it.

Tuesday
3-mile hike, run, walk

Wednesday
Under 100g of carbs

Thursday
200 lateral lunges total

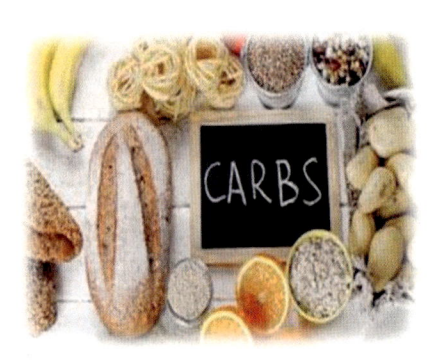

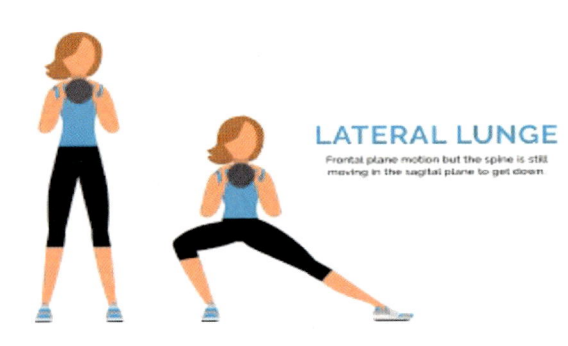

Friday
5 min forward plank
200 sit-ups

Saturday
Yoga, Rom Wod, Mobility

Bonus
Complete 3 plus workouts this week!

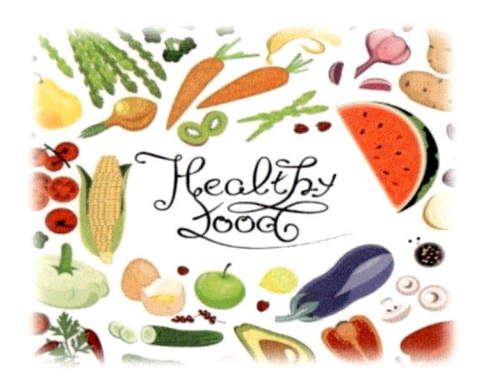

WEEK 3

Monday
100 pushups in addition to your daily workout. Challenge yourself on these. They should be difficult. If you need to modify, drop down to your knees.

Tuesday
Eat the "RAINBOW" today. Each meal consists of 3 foods of different colors of the rainbow. The more color you add, the more micronutrients you consume. Eat color for your health!!

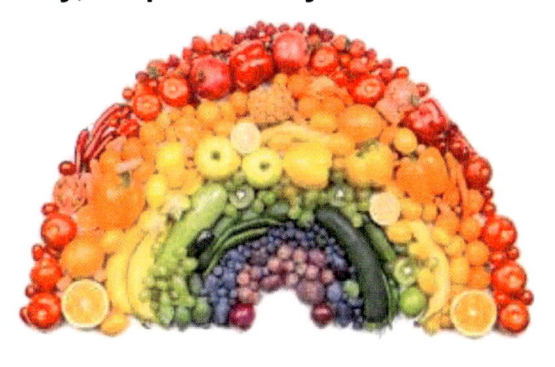

Wednesday
200 4 count flutter kicks and 200 alt v-ups. Core strength is so important for the overall health of your body. If you have a sore back, chances are you need to work on strengthening you core muscles.

Thursday
Limit screen time! Give your mind and eyes a break! Get out and exercise, play a game, other activities other than tv or phone time.

Friday
300 walking lunges in addition to your daily workout. Lunges are excellent for core, leg, glute strength. They also work on mobility.

Saturday
Overall, a healthy lifestyle is about feeling good about yourself. Write down areas that you love about yourself. Three positives about your appearance and three on the type of person you are. Write your strengths and weaknesses.

WEEK 4

Monday
100 additional Kettlebell swings. If you do not have a KB use and object from your home. Ex. water gallon filled; backpack filled with books. Etc.

Tuesday
Low Caffeine intake. No more than 150 mg

Wednesday
Backward walk or run! 5 x 200 m run or brisk walk. This is tough, uses different leg muscles, be careful!

Thursday
Think outside the box and choose a different type of protein then you are used to. Make a new recipe with this.

Friday
Farmers Carry for 800m. Farmers carry, 2 kettlebells or heavy objects held down at your side and you just walk. Focusing on posture and correct form. Keep core engaged. Should be challenging to work your grip strength.

Saturday
Extra reps today! Complete 100 bf sit ups, 50 pushups, and 200 air squats in addition to your daily workout.

Bonus
Accumulate 6 additional miles run or walk throughout the week!

WEEK 5

Monday
Complete 250 Mountain Climbers. Full standards! Start in plank position, drive that knee up as close to that elbow as possible. This exercise is great for core strength and cardio.

Tuesday
Prepare a healthy lunch or dinner. Find a recipe that makes you think outside the box and cook something that is unfamiliar to you. Trying new foods is key to healthy eating.

Wednesday
Get out of the house and participate in 30 plus additional minutes of cardio, your choice. Examples: run, bike, row, swim, hike.

Thursday
No alcohol today. This is especially important when you are looking to lose weight or practice an overall healthier lifestyle.

Friday
5k run for time!!! If you are a runner, try to PR your race time. If you need to modify it for another exercise choose something that is challenging and can be timed.

Saturday
10 rounds
40 sec on 20 sec rest of Burpees
Go hard, keep track of the number of burpees you get each round. Try and stay consistent with that number. Push!!! Modify to a squat thrust if needed!

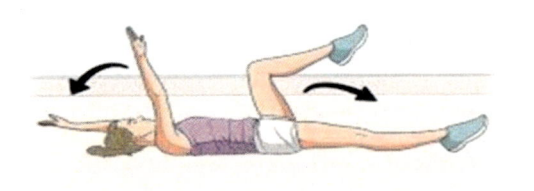

Bonus
20 accumulated minutes of core exercises. Example plank, sit-ups, v ups, straight leg, dead bug.

WEEKLY CHECK IN SHEET AND SCORE

PROGRESS NOTES

WEEK 1

WEEK 2

WEEK 3

WEEK 4

WEEK 5

WEEKLY SCORE

WEEK 1

WEEK 2

WEEK 3

WEEK 4

WEEK 5

CONGRATULATIONS!!!

**You have completed your 5-week challenge to a healthier lifestyle!
Go back to your goals you posted in week 1.
Have you accomplished what you wanted; are there still areas you need improvement on?
Most importantly do not stop all your hard work. Have a healthy relationship with foods and keep up on your workouts. You have 365 of them! You can always go back and repeat to push for heavier weight or PR your times! Be proud of your hard work, be comfortable in your own skin and keep moving!**

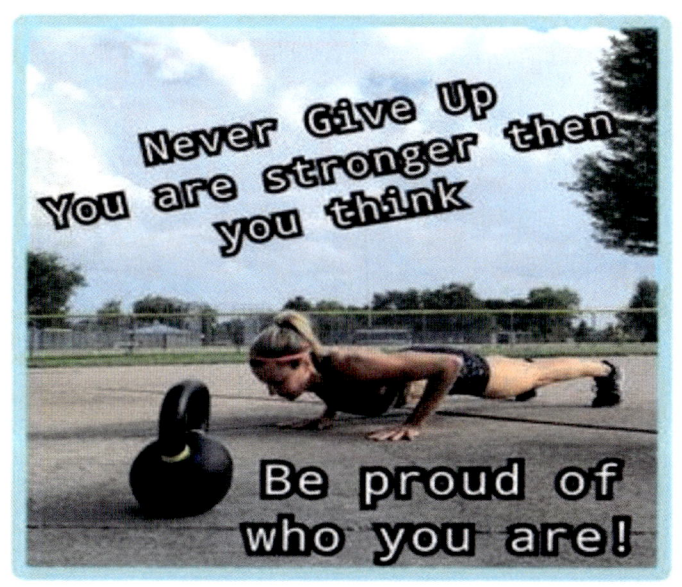

NOTES:

ADVICE FROM THE AUTHOR

Keep in mind that striving for perfection usually leads to disaster. Set small goals and stair step your way to success by developing healthy habits. If it is stressful to change your ways, nutrition, or fitness 100%, start by changing it 50% and eventually working up to your goal!

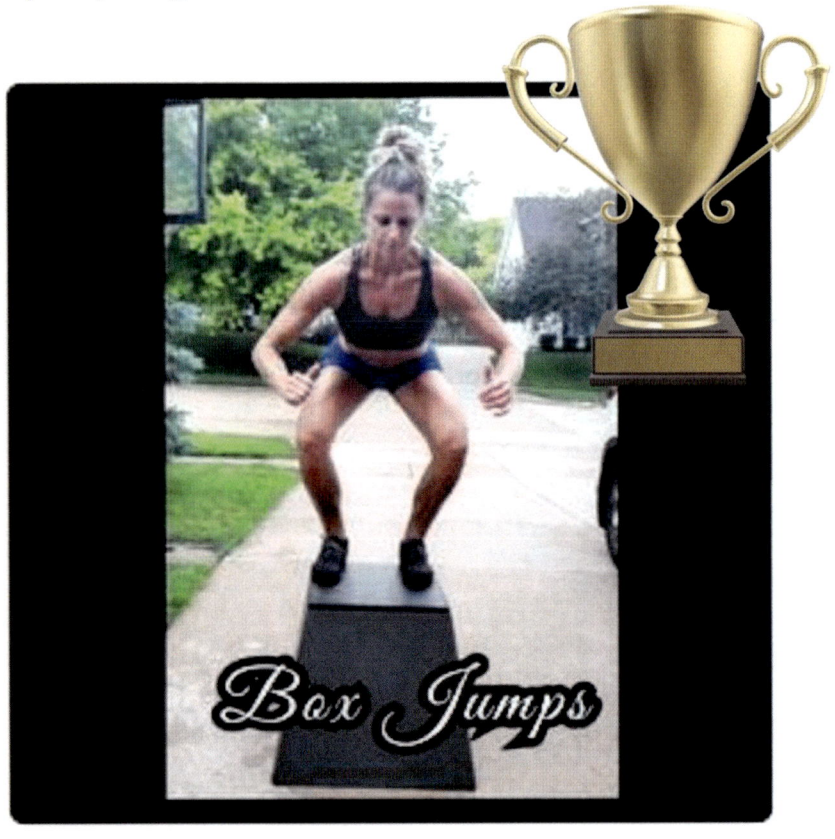

DO NOT DIET Make a liftstyle change towards healthier foods, not a deprivation plan. Find healthy foods you enjoy, new recipes, and join meal prep groups.

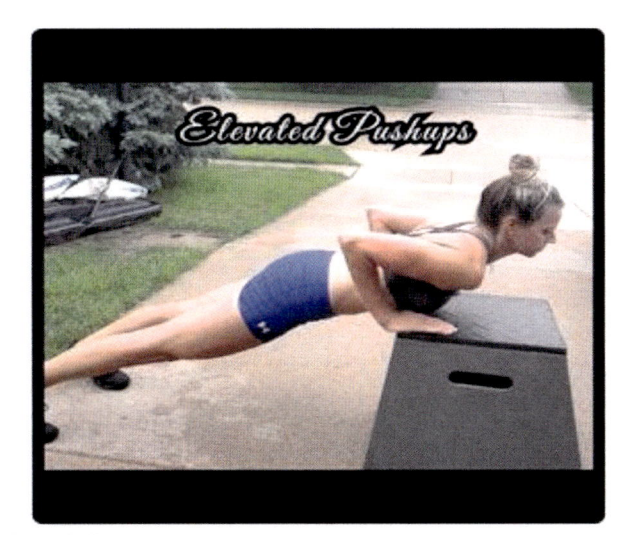

Listen to your Body!

Take Recovery Days, Give yourself one to two days a week for active and mental recovery. This can include taking a walk, gentle yoga class, meditation. Engage in something that's less intense than these workouts.

This is what recovery looks like:

1. Eat balanced and nutritious foods
2. Getting at least 7-9 hours of sleep
3. Drink at least 1 oz of water per lb of body weight a day
4. Listen to your body! Listen to the hints your body gives.

Keep Healthy Snacks on Hand

Select healthier choices to have on standby in your fridge or pantry when hunger pangs or emotional eating strikes, such as nuts, granola, fresh fruit, vegetables, protein shakes, and smoothies.

Keep your journal or fill out the notes section in this book to keep track of the schedule that works for you. It is inspiring for you to look at your successes and keeps you motivated!

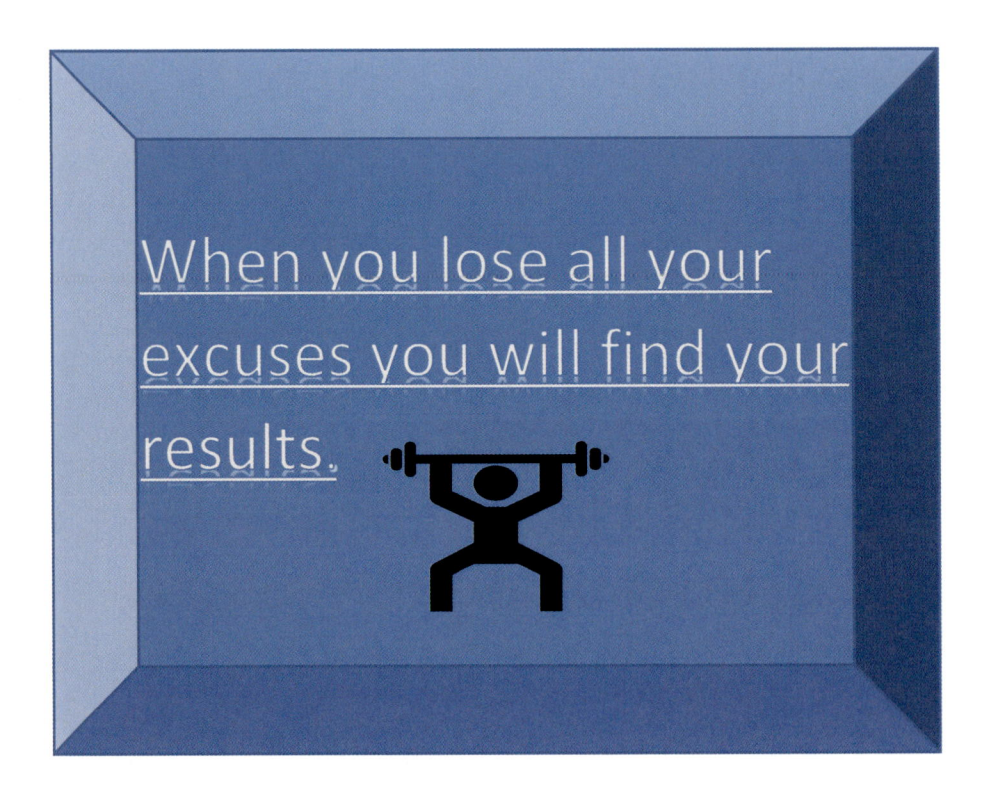

When you lose all your excuses you will find your results.

> Believe in yourself and you'll be unstoppable

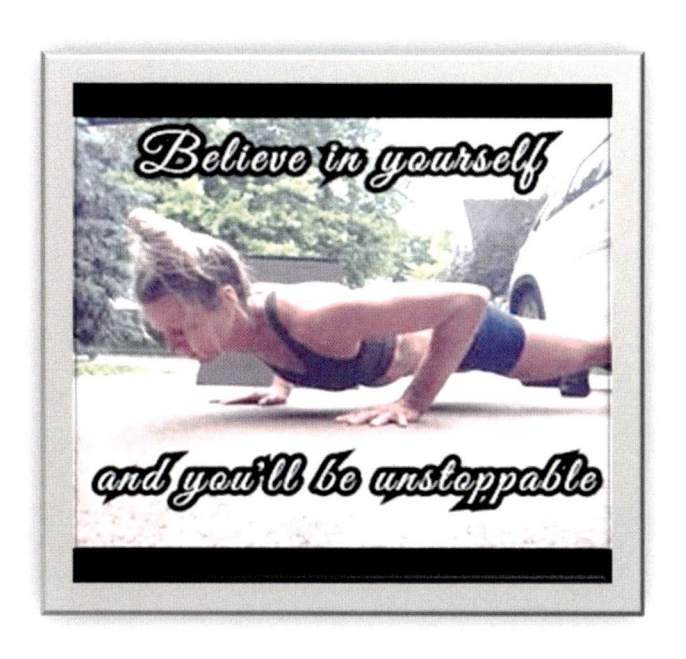

BE PROUD OF YOUR ACCOMPLISHMENTS!!!!
THANK YOU FOR TAKING THIS JOURNEY WITH ME!

You Are Enough!

Made in the USA
Monee, IL
13 December 2020